LISTERIA-FREE LIVING:

A HANDBOOK FOR PREGNANT WOMEN, THE ELDERLY, AND THE IMMUNOCOMPROMISE

Nora Carewell

COPYRIGHT

Copyright © 2024 Nora Carewell

All Rights Reserved

TABLE OF CONTENTS

Preface

Introduction to Listeria-Free Living

Purpose of the Handbook

How to Use This Book

Chapter 1: Understanding Listeria

What is Listeria?

How Listeria Spreads

Symptoms and Health Risks

Why Certain Groups are More Vulnerable

Chapter 2: Listeria and Vulnerable Populations

Risks to Pregnant Women

Risks to the Elderly

Risks to the Immunocompromised

Recognizing Symptoms and Early Detection

Preventative Measures

Chapter 3: Safe Food Practices

General Food Safety Guidelines

Shopping for Safe Food

Storing Food Correctly

Cooking and Reheating Tips

Avoiding Cross-Contamination

Chapter 4: Navigating Food Choices

Foods to Avoid

Safe Alternatives and Substitutes

Understanding Food Labels

Eating Out Safely

Chapter 5: Maintaining a Listeria-Free Home

Kitchen Hygiene and Cleaning

Proper Dishwashing Techniques

Refrigerator and Freezer Maintenance

Handling Leftovers Safely

Chapter 6: Traveling and Listeria Prevention

Preparing for Travel

Safe Eating While Traveling

Managing Food Safety in Different Environments

Emergency Contacts and Resources

Chapter 7: Responding to a Listeria Outbreak and Support

Recognizing a Listeria Outbreak

What to Do if Exposed

Seeking Medical Help

Reporting and Tracking Outbreaks

Support Groups and Communities

Educational Resources

Government and Health Organization Guidelines

Appendices

Glossary of Terms

Frequently Asked Questions

Sample Meal Plans

Contact Information for Health Agencies

Further Reading and References

PREFACE

Welcome to "Listeria-Free Living: A Handbook for Pregnant Women, the Elderly, and the Immunocompromised." This handbook is designed to be a comprehensive guide for those who are particularly vulnerable to Listeria infection. As an author deeply committed to public health, my goal is to provide you with the necessary knowledge and practical advice to protect yourself and your loved ones from this potentially dangerous bacterium.

Listeria monocytogenes is a type of bacteria that can cause serious illness, especially in pregnant women, the elderly, and individuals with weakened immune systems. Understanding how Listeria spreads, recognizing its symptoms, and knowing how to prevent infection are crucial steps in ensuring your health and well-being. This book aims to address these aspects in a clear, straightforward manner.

In writing this handbook, I have drawn upon the latest scientific research, consultations with health experts, and guidelines from reputable health organizations. Each chapter is carefully structured to cover different aspects of Listeria prevention, from food safety practices to recognizing symptoms and responding to outbreaks. Whether you are preparing meals at home, dining out, or traveling, this book offers practical tips and advice to help you make informed decisions.

"Understanding Listeria" introduces you to the nature of the bacterium, how it spreads, and why certain groups are more at risk. "Listeria and Vulnerable Populations" delves into the specific risks and preventative measures for pregnant women, the elderly, and the immunocompromised. "Safe Food Practices" and "Navigating Food Choices" provide detailed guidance on how to handle, store, and prepare food safely, while "Maintaining a Listeria-Free Home" focuses on hygiene practices that can help prevent contamination in your living space. "Traveling and Listeria Prevention" offers advice for staying safe while on the go, and the final chapter, "Responding to a Listeria Outbreak and Support," equips you with the knowledge to handle potential exposures and find support resources.

My hope is that this handbook will serve as a valuable resource in your journey toward a Listeria-free life. The information within these pages is meant to empower you to take proactive steps in safeguarding your health. Thank you for taking the time to read this book, and I wish you and your loved one's good health and peace of mind.

Sincerely,

Nora Carewell.

CHAPTER 1

UNDERSTANDING LISTERIA

What is Listeria?

Listeria monocytogenes, commonly referred to as Listeria, is a type of bacterium that can cause a serious infection known as listeriosis. Unlike many other bacteria, Listeria can thrive in a wide range of environments, including refrigeration temperatures, making it a formidable pathogen. It is particularly concerning because it can survive and multiply even in conditions that typically inhibit the growth of other bacteria.

Listeriosis primarily affects individuals with weakened immune systems, pregnant women, newborns, and the elderly. While healthy adults and children can also become infected, they are generally at a lower risk of severe illness. For those in vulnerable groups, however, listeriosis can lead to severe complications, including septicemia (blood poisoning), meningitis (inflammation of the membranes surrounding the brain and spinal cord), and in the case of pregnant women, miscarriage, stillbirth, or serious infections in newborns.

How Listeria Spreads

Listeria is widely distributed in nature and can be found in soil, water, and animal feces. It can contaminate a variety of foods, including:

- **Raw vegetables**: These can become contaminated from the soil or from manure used as fertilizer.
- **Meat**: Especially undercooked meat.
- **Unpasteurized milk and dairy products**: Listeria can thrive in unpasteurized milk and cheeses.

- **Processed foods**: Such as soft cheeses, deli meats, hot dogs, and smoked seafood.
- **Ready-to-eat foods**: Foods that require no further cooking can be contaminated if they are processed or handled in unhygienic conditions.

Listeria can also spread through cross-contamination, where bacteria from one food item are transferred to another. This can occur through direct contact or indirectly via contaminated surfaces, utensils, or hands. One of the unique characteristics of Listeria is its ability to grow at refrigeration temperatures, which means that even foods stored in the fridge are not completely safe if they become contaminated.

Symptoms and Health Risks

The symptoms of listeriosis can vary widely depending on the individual's overall health and the severity of the infection. Common symptoms include:

- **Fever**
- **Muscle aches**
- **Nausea**
- **Diarrhea**

In more severe cases, particularly in vulnerable populations, symptoms can escalate to:

- **Headache**
- **Stiff neck**
- **Confusion**
- **Loss of balance**
- **Convulsions**

Pregnant women typically experience flu-like symptoms, but the infection can have serious consequences for the fetus, leading to miscarriage, stillbirth, or life-threatening infections in newborns. In older adults and individuals with weakened immune systems, listeriosis can lead to more severe outcomes, including septicemia and meningitis.

Why Certain Groups are More Vulnerable

Certain populations are at greater risk of severe illness from Listeria due to their immune systems' reduced ability to fight off infections. These groups include:

- **Pregnant Women**: During pregnancy, the immune system undergoes changes to protect the fetus, making pregnant women more susceptible to infections. Listeriosis can cross the placenta, infecting the fetus and potentially leading to miscarriage, stillbirth, or neonatal infections.

- **Newborns**: Infants' immune systems are not fully developed, making them more vulnerable to severe infections.
- **Elderly Individuals**: Aging can weaken the immune system, and older adults are more likely to have underlying health conditions that make them susceptible to infections.
- **Immunocompromised Individuals**: People with weakened immune systems, whether due to diseases such as HIV/AIDS, cancer, diabetes, or treatments like chemotherapy or immunosuppressive drugs, are at a higher risk of contracting and suffering severe consequences from listeriosis.

Historical Context and Notable Outbreaks

Understanding the history of Listeria and notable outbreaks can shed light on its impact and the importance of prevention measures. One of the most significant outbreaks occurred in Canada in 2008, linked to contaminated deli meats produced by Maple Leaf Foods. This outbreak resulted in 57 confirmed cases and 23 deaths, highlighting the bacterium's lethal potential.

Another major outbreak took place in the United States in 2011, traced to cantaloupes from Jensen Farms in Colorado. This outbreak led to 147 cases and 33 deaths, making it one of the deadliest foodborne outbreaks in U.S. history. These and other outbreaks underscore the need for stringent food safety practices and vigilant monitoring to prevent contamination.

The Lifecycle of Listeria

Listeria has a unique lifecycle that enables it to survive and thrive in various environments. It can exist as a saprophyte in soil, where it feeds on decaying organic matter, or as a pathogen in animal and human hosts. Its ability to adapt to different conditions, including low temperatures and high salt concentrations, makes it particularly resilient.

Listeria's lifecycle includes:

1. **Entry and Colonization**: Listeria enters the body through ingestion of contaminated food. It then colonizes the intestines, where it can invade the intestinal lining and spread to other parts of the body.
2. **Intracellular Survival**: Listeria has the ability to invade and survive within host cells, evading the immune system. It can move from cell to cell, spreading the infection while avoiding detection.
3. **Systemic Spread**: From the intestines, Listeria can enter the

bloodstream, leading to septicemia, and cross the blood-brain barrier to cause meningitis. In pregnant women, it can cross the placenta and infect the fetus.

Diagnosis and Treatment

Diagnosing listeriosis can be challenging, as its symptoms often resemble those of other illnesses. If listeriosis is suspected, doctors typically use blood tests, spinal fluid tests, or tests of amniotic fluid or the placenta to confirm the presence of Listeria.

Treatment for listeriosis typically involves antibiotics, with the choice of antibiotic depending on the severity of the infection and the patient's overall health. Common antibiotics used include ampicillin and gentamicin. Early diagnosis and treatment are crucial, especially for pregnant women and individuals with weakened immune systems, to prevent severe complications.

Preventing Listeria Infection

Prevention is the most effective way to combat listeriosis, particularly for those in high-risk groups. Key preventive measures include:

- **Practicing Good Hygiene**: Washing hands thoroughly with soap and water before and after handling food, as well as after using the bathroom, changing diapers, or touching animals.
- **Safe Food Handling**: Keeping raw meat separate from other foods, using separate cutting boards for raw meat and other foods, and ensuring that all utensils and surfaces are thoroughly cleaned.
- **Proper Cooking and Storage**: Cooking meat and poultry to safe temperatures, promptly refrigerating

leftovers, and avoiding unpasteurized dairy products.
- **Vigilance with Ready-to-Eat Foods**: Being cautious with deli meats, hot dogs, and other ready-to-eat foods, which should be heated until steaming hot before consumption, especially for pregnant women and individuals with weakened immune systems.

CHAPTER 2

LISTERIA AND VULNERABLE POPULATIONS

Introduction

Listeria monocytogenes poses a significant health threat to certain populations, including pregnant women, the elderly, and individuals with weakened immune systems. This chapter delves into the unique risks and challenges faced by these vulnerable groups, providing detailed information on symptoms, preventative measures, and specific guidelines to help mitigate the risk of listeriosis.

Risks to Pregnant Women

Pregnancy brings about significant changes in a woman's body, including alterations to the immune system that can increase susceptibility to infections like listeriosis. Pregnant women are about ten times more likely to get listeriosis compared to the general population. This increased risk is due to the immune system's natural adaptation to protect the developing fetus, which inadvertently makes it less effective at warding off certain infections.

Impact on Pregnancy and Fetal Health

Listeriosis during pregnancy can have severe consequences for both the mother and the fetus. While pregnant women might experience only mild flu-like symptoms, the infection can cross the placenta and lead to serious complications such as:

- **Miscarriage**: Listeriosis can cause early pregnancy loss.
- **Stillbirth**: The infection can lead to fetal death later in pregnancy.

- **Preterm Labor**: Listeriosis can induce premature labor, which carries its own set of risks for the baby.
- **Neonatal Infection**: Babies born with listeriosis can suffer from severe infections, including sepsis and meningitis, which can be life-threatening.

Symptoms in Pregnant Women

The symptoms of listeriosis in pregnant women can be non-specific and resemble those of a mild flu or a gastrointestinal illness. Common symptoms include:

- Fever
- Muscle aches
- Fatigue
- Nausea and vomiting
- Diarrhea

Given the potential severity of the infection, it is crucial for pregnant women to seek medical attention if they experience these symptoms, particularly if they have consumed high-risk foods.

Preventative Measures for Pregnant Women

Preventing listeriosis is especially important during pregnancy. Here are key strategies:

- **Avoid High-Risk Foods**: Pregnant women should avoid certain foods that are more likely to be contaminated with Listeria. These include unpasteurized dairy products, soft cheeses (such as feta, brie, and blue cheese), deli meats, hot dogs, and smoked seafood unless they are cooked until steaming hot.
- **Practice Safe Food Handling**: Wash hands, utensils, and food

preparation surfaces thoroughly before and after handling food. Keep raw meats separate from other foods.

- **Cook Foods Thoroughly**: Ensure that meats, poultry, and seafood are cooked to safe internal temperatures. Use a food thermometer to check doneness.
- **Refrigerate Promptly**: Store leftovers in the refrigerator promptly and consume them within a few days. Ensure that your refrigerator is set to 40°F (4°C) or lower and your freezer to 0°F (-18°C) or lower.
- **Be Cautious with Ready-to-Eat Foods**: Heat deli meats and hot dogs until steaming hot before consuming.

Risks to the Elderly

As people age, their immune systems naturally weaken, making them more susceptible to infections. The elderly population is at increased risk for severe illness from listeriosis due to this decline in immune function and the higher likelihood of having underlying health conditions.

Health Implications for the Elderly

Listeriosis in the elderly can lead to serious health complications, including:

- **Septicemia**: Bloodstream infection that can cause severe illness and even death.
- **Meningitis**: Inflammation of the membranes surrounding the brain and spinal cord, which can be life-threatening.
- **Endocarditis**: Infection of the inner lining of the heart chambers and valves, which is a rare but serious complication.

Symptoms in the Elderly

The symptoms of listeriosis in older adults can vary but often include:

- Fever
- Muscle aches
- Headache
- Stiff neck
- Confusion or changes in mental status
- Loss of balance
- Convulsions

Because these symptoms can be mistaken for other illnesses, it is important for elderly individuals and their caregivers to be aware of the potential for listeriosis, especially if they have consumed high-risk foods.

Preventative Measures for the Elderly

Elderly individuals can reduce their risk of listeriosis by following these guidelines:

- **Maintain Good Hygiene**: Wash hands regularly, especially before and after handling food.
- **Safe Food Preparation**: Use separate cutting boards for raw meat and other foods, and ensure that all utensils and surfaces are cleaned thoroughly.
- **Cook Foods Properly**: Use a food thermometer to ensure that meats, poultry, and seafood are cooked to safe temperatures.
- **Avoid High-Risk Foods**: Stay away from unpasteurized dairy products, soft cheeses, deli meats, and smoked seafood unless heated until steaming hot.
- **Refrigerate Foods Promptly**: Store leftovers in the refrigerator promptly and consume them within a few days. Ensure that the refrigerator is set to the correct temperature.

Risks to the Immunocompromised

Individuals with weakened immune systems, whether due to medical conditions or treatments, are at a higher risk for listeriosis. This group includes people with HIV/AIDS, cancer patients undergoing chemotherapy, organ transplant recipients on immunosuppressive drugs, and those with chronic illnesses such as diabetes.

Health Implications for the Immunocompromised

Listeriosis in immunocompromised individuals can lead to severe and potentially fatal infections. Complications include:

- **Septicemia**: A serious bloodstream infection that can quickly become life-threatening.

- **Meningitis**: Infection and inflammation of the membranes surrounding the brain and spinal cord.
- **Encephalitis**: Inflammation of the brain itself, which can result in severe neurological damage.
- **Endocarditis**: Infection of the heart valves.

Symptoms in the Immunocompromised

The symptoms of listeriosis in immunocompromised individuals can be severe and may include:

- High fever
- Severe muscle aches
- Headache
- Stiff neck
- Confusion or changes in mental status
- Loss of balance

- Convulsions

Due to the high risk of severe illness, it is crucial for immunocompromised individuals to seek medical attention immediately if they experience these symptoms, particularly if they have consumed high-risk foods.

Preventative Measures for the Immunocompromised

Preventing listeriosis in immunocompromised individuals involves stringent food safety practices:

- **Avoid High-Risk Foods**: Refrain from consuming unpasteurized dairy products, soft cheeses, deli meats, hot dogs, and smoked seafood unless they are thoroughly heated.
- **Practice Good Hygiene**: Wash hands thoroughly with soap and water before and after handling food.

- **Safe Food Handling**: Keep raw meats separate from other foods, and use separate cutting boards for raw and cooked foods.
- **Cook Foods Properly**: Ensure that all meats, poultry, and seafood are cooked to safe temperatures using a food thermometer.
- **Refrigerate Foods Promptly**: Store leftovers in the refrigerator promptly and consume them within a few days. Ensure that the refrigerator is set to the correct temperature.

Recognizing Symptoms and Early Detection

Early detection of listeriosis is crucial for effective treatment, particularly in vulnerable populations. Recognizing the symptoms and seeking medical attention promptly can significantly improve outcomes.

Symptoms Overview

- **Flu-like Symptoms**: Fever, muscle aches, fatigue, and gastrointestinal symptoms such as nausea and diarrhea.
- **Severe Symptoms**: Headache, stiff neck, confusion, loss of balance, and convulsions.

When to Seek Medical Attention

Individuals in high-risk groups should seek medical attention if they experience any of the following:

- Flu-like symptoms after consuming high-risk foods
- Severe headache and stiff neck
- Changes in mental status or confusion
- Loss of balance or convulsions

Medical professionals can perform tests to confirm the presence of Listeria, such as blood tests, spinal fluid tests, or tests of amniotic fluid or the placenta in pregnant women.

CHAPTER 3

SAFE FOOD PRACTICES TO PREVENT LISTERIOSIS

Introduction

Preventing listeriosis, especially among vulnerable populations, hinges on adopting meticulous food safety practices. This chapter provides an in-depth guide on safe food handling, preparation, and storage practices to minimize the risk of Listeria contamination. By implementing these measures, individuals can significantly reduce their chances of contracting this serious infection.

Understanding Food Contamination

Food contamination can occur at any stage from farm to table. Understanding how contamination happens helps in identifying critical points where food safety practices can be applied effectively.

Sources of Contamination

Raw Ingredients: Listeria can be present in raw meats, dairy products, and produce.

Processing: Contamination can occur during processing if hygiene practices are not followed.

Storage and Transport: Improper storage temperatures and handling can lead to bacterial growth.

Preparation and Cooking: Cross-contamination from raw to cooked foods or improper cooking temperatures can allow bacteria to survive.

Shopping for Safe Foods

Preventing listeriosis starts with careful selection of food products. Here are some tips for shopping safely:

Choosing Fresh and Safe Products

Dairy and Eggs:

Select only pasteurized dairy products.
Check expiration dates on all dairy and egg products.
Avoid soft cheeses unless labeled as made with pasteurized milk.

Meats and Seafood:

Choose fresh meats and seafood from reputable sources.
Avoid pre-packaged deli meats and smoked seafood unless cooked.

Produce:

Select fresh, undamaged fruits and vegetables.
Avoid pre-cut or pre-packaged produce unless certain of the safety standards of the supplier.

Prepared and Ready-to-Eat Foods:

Ensure that ready-to-eat foods are stored at proper temperatures in the store.
Avoid items from salad bars or buffets if unsure about the hygiene practices.

Packaging and Handling

Check Packaging:

Avoid products with damaged or bulging packaging.
Ensure vacuum-sealed packages are intact.

Separate Raw and Ready-to-Eat Foods:

Use separate bags for raw meats and ready-to-eat foods to prevent cross-contamination.

Timely Shopping:

Plan your shopping trip so that perishable items are purchased last and transported home quickly.

Safe Food Storage

Proper storage is crucial to prevent the growth of Listeria. This section covers best practices for storing different types of food.

Refrigeration and Freezing

Refrigerator Settings:

Keep the refrigerator temperature at 40°F (4°C) or below.
Use a refrigerator thermometer to monitor the temperature.

Freezer Settings:

Keep the freezer temperature at 0°F (-18°C) or below.
Use a freezer thermometer to monitor the temperature.

Storing Raw Meats and Seafood:

Store raw meats and seafood on the bottom shelf of the refrigerator to prevent juices from dripping onto other foods.

Use sealed containers or plastic bags to contain any leaks.

Storing Dairy and Eggs:

Keep dairy products and eggs in their original containers.

Store eggs in the main body of the refrigerator, not the door, to maintain a consistent temperature.

Storing Produce:

Refrigerate perishable fruits and vegetables. Store leafy greens and herbs in airtight containers or plastic bags to maintain freshness.

Leftovers and Prepared Foods:

Store leftovers in airtight containers.

Label containers with the date to keep track of their freshness.

Safe Food Preparation

Proper food preparation techniques are essential in preventing listeriosis. This section outlines the steps to take to ensure safe preparation of meals.

Washing Hands and Surfaces

Hand Washing:

Wash hands with soap and water for at least 20 seconds before and after handling food.
Wash hands after using the restroom, handling pets, and changing diapers.

Cleaning Surfaces and Utensils:

Clean countertops, cutting boards, and utensils with hot, soapy water before and after preparing food.

Use separate cutting boards for raw meats and other foods to prevent cross-contamination.

Sanitize surfaces and utensils regularly, especially after contact with raw meat, poultry, or seafood.

Washing Produce

Fruits and Vegetables:

Rinse all fruits and vegetables under running water before eating, cutting, or cooking.

Use a brush to scrub firm produce like melons and cucumbers.

Dry produce with a clean cloth or paper towel to remove any remaining bacteria.

Safe Thawing Practices

Refrigerator Thawing:

Thaw frozen meats and seafood in the refrigerator, not on the countertop.

Place thawing items on a plate or in a container to catch any drips.

Cold Water Thawing:

For quicker thawing, place frozen food in a sealed plastic bag and submerge it in cold water.

Change the water every 30 minutes to keep it cold.

Microwave Thawing:

Thaw food in the microwave if planning to cook it immediately afterward.

Cooking to Safe Temperatures

Using a Food Thermometer:

Use a food thermometer to ensure meats, poultry, and seafood are cooked to safe internal temperatures.

Insert the thermometer into the thickest part of the food, avoiding bone or fat.

Safe Cooking Temperatures:

Poultry (whole, parts, and ground): 165°F (74°C)

Ground meats (beef, pork, lamb, and veal): 160°F (71°C)

Beef, pork, lamb, and veal (steaks, chops, roasts): 145°F (63°C) with a three-minute rest time

Fish and shellfish: 145°F (63°C)

Safe Food Serving

Once food is prepared safely, it is important to serve it in a way that maintains its safety.

Serving Hot Foods

Keep Foods Hot:

Maintain hot foods at 140°F (60°C) or above until serving.
Use chafing dishes, slow cookers, and warming trays to keep food hot.

Stirring Foods:

Stir foods occasionally to ensure even heating.

Serving Cold Foods

Keep Foods Cold:

Maintain cold foods at 40°F (4°C) or below. Use ice or cold packs to keep foods cold at buffets or picnics.

Serving in Small Portions:

Serve food in smaller portions and replenish from the refrigerator as needed to keep food at safe temperatures.

Safe Food Storage After Serving

Leftovers can pose a risk if not handled properly. Follow these guidelines to store leftovers safely.

Cooling Leftovers

Prompt Refrigeration:

Refrigerate leftovers within two hours of cooking or serving.
In hot weather (above 90°F or 32°C), refrigerate within one hour.

Shallow Containers:

Store leftovers in shallow containers to cool quickly and evenly.

Reheating Leftovers

Reheat to Safe Temperatures:

Reheat leftovers to an internal temperature of 165°F (74°C).
Use a food thermometer to check the temperature.

Microwave Reheating:

When reheating in a microwave, cover food and rotate or stir it halfway through heating to ensure even heating.

Avoiding Recontamination:

Only reheat the portion of food that will be consumed.
Avoid reheating food more than once.

Special Considerations for Vulnerable Populations

Vulnerable populations need to be extra vigilant in their food safety practices. This section highlights additional precautions for pregnant women, the elderly, and immunocompromised individuals.

Pregnant Women

Avoiding High-Risk Foods:

Do not consume unpasteurized dairy products, raw or undercooked meats, and smoked seafood unless heated until steaming hot.
Avoid ready-to-eat deli meats and hot dogs unless they are reheated to steaming hot.

Maintaining Cleanliness:

Wash hands and surfaces thoroughly to avoid cross-contamination.
Be cautious with leftovers and ready-to-eat foods.

The Elderly

Careful Food Selection:

Choose pasteurized dairy products and avoid high-risk foods.
Ensure all meats and seafood are cooked to safe internal temperatures.

Safe Food Storage:

Refrigerate perishable foods promptly and keep track of expiration dates.
Avoid consuming foods past their expiration dates.

Immunocompromised Individuals

Avoiding Contaminated Foods:

Avoid high-risk foods such as unpasteurized dairy products, raw or undercooked meats, and smoked seafood.
Be cautious with raw fruits and vegetables; consider cooking them to reduce the risk of contamination.

Maintaining a Clean Environment:

Wash hands, surfaces, and utensils thoroughly before and after food preparation.

Use separate cutting boards for raw and cooked foods to prevent cross-contamination.

Monitoring and Managing Food Safety at Home

Ongoing vigilance is required to maintain food safety at home. This section outlines strategies for monitoring and managing food safety practices.

Regular Kitchen Inspections

Check for Cleanliness:

Regularly clean and sanitize kitchen surfaces, including countertops, cutting boards, and sinks.

Ensure that all utensils and appliances are clean and in good working condition.

Inspect Food Storage Areas:

Regularly check the refrigerator and freezer for proper temperatures.
Ensure that food is stored in airtight containers to prevent contamination.

Food Safety Education

Stay Informed:

Keep up-to-date with food safety guidelines and recalls from reliable sources such as the CDC and FDA.
Educate family members and others involved in food preparation about safe food handling practices.

Food Safety Tools:

Use tools such as refrigerator thermometers and food thermometers to monitor food safety.

Implement food safety checklists to ensure that all steps are followed during food preparation and storage.

CHAPTER 4

IDENTIFYING AND MANAGING SYMPTOMS OF LISTERIOSIS

Introduction

Listeriosis is a serious infection caused by eating food contaminated with the bacterium Listeria monocytogenes. While healthy individuals may experience mild symptoms, certain groups, including pregnant women, newborns, the elderly, and immunocompromised individuals, are at a higher risk of severe illness. This chapter delves into the symptoms of listeriosis, how to recognize them, and the steps to manage and seek treatment for the infection.

Recognizing the Symptoms of Listeriosis

Listeriosis can present a range of symptoms depending on the individual's health status and the infection's progression. Early recognition of symptoms is crucial for timely treatment.

General Symptoms

Fever and Muscle Aches: Most people with listeriosis experience flu-like symptoms such as fever and muscle aches.

Gastrointestinal Symptoms: Diarrhea, nausea, and vomiting may occur in some individuals.

Headache and Stiff Neck: As the infection progresses, individuals may experience headaches and a stiff neck, which can indicate meningitis.

Confusion and Loss of Balance: Severe cases may lead to confusion and loss of balance due to the bacteria spreading to the nervous system.

Symptoms in Pregnant Women

Flu-like Symptoms: Pregnant women often experience mild, flu-like symptoms such as fever, fatigue, and muscle aches.

Pregnancy Complications: Listeriosis during pregnancy can lead to serious complications including miscarriage, stillbirth, premature delivery, or life-threatening infection of the newborn.

Symptoms in Newborns

Sepsis: Newborns infected with listeriosis may develop sepsis, characterized by fever, difficulty feeding, irritability, and lethargy.

Respiratory Distress: Difficulty breathing and other respiratory issues may occur.

Meningitis: Newborns can develop meningitis, leading to symptoms such as a bulging fontanel (soft spot on the head), stiffness, and seizures.

Symptoms in the Elderly and Immunocompromised

Severe Illness: These groups are more likely to experience severe symptoms, including septicemia and meningitis.
Neurological Symptoms: Confusion, loss of balance, and convulsions are common in severe cases.

When to Seek Medical Attention

Prompt medical attention is essential when listeriosis is suspected, especially for those in high-risk groups. Early treatment can prevent complications and improve outcomes.

Recognizing the Need for Medical Help

Persistent Fever and Muscle Aches: If flu-like symptoms persist for more than a few days or worsen, seek medical attention.

Gastrointestinal Distress: Severe or prolonged diarrhea, nausea, or vomiting should not be ignored.

Neurological Symptoms: Headache, stiff neck, confusion, or loss of balance warrant immediate medical evaluation.

Pregnancy Concerns: Pregnant women experiencing fever and other symptoms should seek prompt medical care to protect themselves and their unborn child.

What to Expect During a Medical Visit

Medical History and Symptoms: The healthcare provider will take a detailed medical history and ask about symptoms, including any recent food consumption that may have been contaminated.

Physical Examination: A physical exam will be conducted to assess the severity of symptoms and identify any signs of neurological involvement.

Diagnostic Tests: Blood tests, lumbar puncture (spinal tap), and imaging studies may be ordered to confirm the diagnosis and determine the extent of the infection.

Diagnosing Listeriosis

Accurate diagnosis is critical for effective treatment. Several tests and procedures can help confirm listeriosis.

Laboratory Tests

Blood Cultures: Blood samples are taken to detect the presence of Listeria bacteria.

CSF Analysis: If meningitis is suspected, a lumbar puncture is performed to obtain cerebrospinal fluid (CSF) for analysis.

Stool Samples: In some cases, stool samples may be tested for Listeria, especially if gastrointestinal symptoms are prominent.

Imaging Studies

MRI and CT Scans: Imaging studies of the brain may be conducted to assess for signs of meningitis or abscesses.

Ultrasound: For pregnant women, ultrasound can help monitor the health of the fetus and detect any complications.

Treatment of Listeriosis

Treatment for listeriosis typically involves antibiotics, but the approach may vary depending on the patient's health status and the severity of the infection.

Antibiotic Therapy

Common Antibiotics: Ampicillin and gentamicin are commonly used to treat listeriosis. These antibiotics are usually administered intravenously in a hospital setting.

Treatment Duration: The duration of antibiotic therapy can vary from two weeks to several months, depending on the severity of the infection and the patient's response to treatment.

Supportive Care

Hospitalization: Severe cases, especially those involving septicemia or meningitis, often require hospitalization for close monitoring and intensive care.

Hydration and Nutrition: Ensuring adequate hydration and nutrition is vital, particularly for those experiencing gastrointestinal symptoms.

Special Considerations for Vulnerable Populations

Pregnant Women: Antibiotic treatment is essential to prevent complications for both mother and baby. Early intervention can significantly reduce the risk of miscarriage, stillbirth, or neonatal infection.

Newborns: Infected newborns require prompt antibiotic treatment and may need supportive care in a neonatal intensive care unit (NICU).

Elderly and Immunocompromised: These patients may need longer courses of antibiotics and more intensive supportive care due to their weakened immune systems.

Managing Symptoms at Home

While some cases of listeriosis require hospitalization, mild cases can be managed at home with appropriate care and monitoring.

Symptom Relief

Fever and Pain Management: Over-the-counter medications such as acetaminophen or ibuprofen can help reduce fever and alleviate muscle aches and pain.

Hydration: Staying well-hydrated is crucial, especially if experiencing diarrhea or vomiting. Oral rehydration solutions can help maintain electrolyte balance.

Rest: Adequate rest is essential to support the body's immune response and recovery.

Monitoring Symptoms

Temperature Monitoring: Regularly check body temperature to ensure fever is under control.

Watch for Worsening Symptoms: Be vigilant for signs of worsening illness, such as increased fever, persistent vomiting, severe headache, or neurological symptoms, and seek medical attention if they occur.

Nutrition and Diet

Easy-to-Digest Foods: Consume easy-to-digest foods like soups, broths, and plain rice to avoid further gastrointestinal distress.

Avoid High-Risk Foods: Continue to avoid foods that may be contaminated with Listeria, such as unpasteurized dairy products, deli meats, and certain seafood.

Preventing Recurrence

After recovering from listeriosis, it is important to take steps to prevent a recurrence. This involves ongoing vigilance in food safety practices and regular health check-ups.

Continued Food Safety Practices

Adhere to Safe Food Handling: Follow the food safety guidelines discussed in Chapter 3 to minimize the risk of re-infection.

Educate Household Members: Ensure that everyone in the household is aware of safe food handling practices to prevent contamination.

Regular Health Monitoring

Follow-Up Medical Visits: Schedule follow-up visits with your healthcare provider to monitor your recovery and address any lingering health concerns.

Health Screenings: Regular health screenings can help detect any underlying conditions that may increase the risk of listeriosis or other infections.

Supporting Loved Ones

If a family member or friend is diagnosed with listeriosis, offering support and assistance can be invaluable. This section provides tips on how to help loved ones manage their illness and recovery.

Providing Emotional Support

Be Understanding and Compassionate: Listeriosis can be a stressful and frightening experience, especially for vulnerable individuals. Offer empathy and understanding.

Encourage Communication: Encourage your loved one to express their feelings and concerns about their illness and recovery.

Assisting with Daily Activities

Help with Food Preparation: Assist with preparing safe and nutritious meals, following food safety guidelines to prevent contamination.

Transportation to Medical Appointments: Offer to drive your loved one to medical appointments and help them navigate the healthcare system.

Monitoring Symptoms

Watch for Warning Signs: Be vigilant for any signs of worsening illness and seek medical attention if necessary.

Encourage Medication Adherence: Remind your loved one to take prescribed medications as directed and complete the full course of antibiotics.

Listeriosis and Long-Term Health

Recovering from listeriosis is an important milestone, but it is also essential to consider the long-term health implications. This section explores how to maintain overall health and prevent future infections.

Strengthening the Immune System

Balanced Diet: Eat a balanced diet rich in fruits, vegetables, lean proteins, and whole grains to support immune function.

Regular Exercise: Engage in regular physical activity to boost overall health and strengthen the immune system.

Adequate Sleep: Ensure you get enough restful sleep each night to support immune function and overall well-being.

Managing Chronic Conditions

Follow Medical Advice: Adhere to treatment plans and follow medical advice for managing any chronic conditions, such as diabetes or heart disease.

Regular Check-Ups: Schedule regular check-ups with your healthcare provider to monitor your health and address any emerging issues.

Chapter 5

PREVENTING LISTERIOSIS IN HIGH-RISK GROUPS

Introduction

Listeriosis is a significant health concern, especially for those in high-risk groups, including pregnant women, the elderly, and individuals with compromised immune systems. Prevention is crucial for these groups to avoid the severe consequences associated with Listeria monocytogenes infections. This chapter focuses on practical strategies to prevent listeriosis, emphasizing food safety, lifestyle adjustments, and health monitoring specific to high-risk populations.

Food Safety Practices

Food safety is the cornerstone of preventing listeriosis. Adhering to rigorous food safety practices can significantly reduce the risk of infection.

Safe Food Handling

Washing Hands: Proper hand hygiene is essential. Wash hands thoroughly with soap and water before and after handling food, especially raw meats, seafood, and vegetables.

Cleaning Surfaces: Ensure that all kitchen surfaces, including countertops, cutting boards, and utensils, are cleaned and sanitized regularly. Use hot, soapy water and a disinfectant suitable for kitchen use.

Avoid Cross-Contamination: Use separate cutting boards and utensils for raw meats and other food items to prevent cross-contamination. Store raw meats separately in the refrigerator, ideally on the bottom shelf to avoid dripping onto other foods.

Safe Food Preparation

Cooking Temperatures: Cook meats, poultry, and seafood to the recommended internal temperatures to kill harmful bacteria. For example, poultry should reach an internal temperature of 165°F (74°C), and ground meats should reach 160°F (71°C).

Refrigeration: Keep your refrigerator at or below 40°F (4°C) and your freezer at 0°F (-18°C). These temperatures inhibit the growth of Listeria monocytogenes and other pathogens.

Food Storage: Store perishable foods, including leftovers, in airtight containers. Consume leftovers within a few days or freeze them for longer storage.

Special Considerations for High-Risk Groups

Pregnant Women: Pregnant women should avoid high-risk foods such as unpasteurized dairy products, deli meats, and soft cheeses. These foods are more likely to be contaminated with Listeria monocytogenes.

Elderly and Immunocompromised: For these groups, avoiding raw or undercooked foods, including unpasteurized dairy products, and ensuring thorough cooking of all meats is particularly important.

Safe Food Choices

Choosing foods that are less likely to harbor Listeria monocytogenes is a vital part of prevention.

Avoiding High-Risk Foods

Unpasteurized Products: Avoid unpasteurized milk and cheese, which can harbor Listeria monocytogenes. Always choose pasteurized products.

Ready-to-Eat Meats: Deli meats, hot dogs, and pâtés should be heated until steaming hot before consumption to kill any potential bacteria.

Soft Cheeses: Soft cheeses, such as feta, brie, and camembert, should be avoided unless they are made from pasteurized milk.

Selecting Safe Alternatives

Fruits and Vegetables: Wash fruits and vegetables thoroughly under running water before eating or cooking. Use a brush for produce with hard surfaces.

Cooked Foods: Choose freshly cooked foods over processed or pre-packaged meals. If consuming leftovers, ensure they are reheated thoroughly to a temperature of at least 165°F (74°C).

Lifestyle Adjustments for High-Risk Groups

Making lifestyle changes can further reduce the risk of listeriosis. This includes adopting habits that support overall health and minimize exposure to infection.

Personal Hygiene

Handwashing: Practice good hand hygiene consistently, especially after using the restroom, before eating, and after handling raw food.
Clean Clothing: Wear clean clothing and use clean dish towels and cloths in the kitchen to prevent contamination.

Health Monitoring

Regular Check-Ups: Regular medical check-ups are crucial for high-risk individuals. Monitoring health can help detect any early signs of infection or complications.

Immunizations: Stay up-to-date with recommended vaccinations, which can help bolster the immune system and reduce the risk of infections.

Health Education and Awareness

Educating high-risk groups about listeriosis and its prevention is critical for reducing incidence rates. Awareness campaigns and educational resources play a significant role.

Community Programs

Health Workshops: Participate in community health workshops that focus on food safety and listeriosis prevention. These workshops can provide valuable information and practical tips.

Support Groups: Join support groups for pregnant women, elderly individuals, or those with compromised immune systems to share experiences and receive support.

Educational Materials

Printed Guides: Use educational brochures, flyers, and booklets that provide information on preventing listeriosis. Distribute these materials through healthcare providers, community centers, and schools.

Online Resources: Access reputable online resources, such as those provided by the CDC and FDA, to stay informed about food safety guidelines and updates on listeriosis prevention.

Food Safety Tools and Technology

Utilizing tools and technology can enhance food safety practices and help prevent listeriosis.

Kitchen Tools

Thermometers: Use food thermometers to ensure that meats and other foods are cooked to the appropriate temperatures.

Refrigerator Thermometers: Place thermometers in your refrigerator and freezer to monitor and maintain safe temperatures.

Technology and Apps

Food Safety Apps: Utilize mobile apps that offer food safety tips, recall alerts, and temperature monitoring features.

Online Food Safety Resources: Access online resources for real-time updates on food recalls, safety guidelines, and educational materials.

Managing Risk During Pregnancy

Pregnant women are at a higher risk for listeriosis, making it essential to adopt specific preventive measures to protect both themselves and their unborn children.

Dietary Restrictions

Avoid High-Risk Foods: Completely avoid unpasteurized dairy products, undercooked meats, and ready-to-eat deli meats unless they are heated to steaming hot.

Safe Cooking Practices: Ensure that all foods are thoroughly cooked, including meats, eggs, and seafood, to eliminate any risk of contamination.

Prenatal Care

Regular Check-Ups: Attend all scheduled prenatal appointments and discuss any concerns related to food safety and listeriosis with your healthcare provider.

Health Monitoring: Monitor any symptoms of illness and seek medical attention promptly if symptoms such as fever, muscle aches, or gastrointestinal distress occur.

Preventing Listeriosis in the Elderly

The elderly are particularly vulnerable to severe cases of listeriosis. Implementing preventive measures is crucial for reducing their risk.

Nutrition and Diet

Balanced Diet: Ensure a balanced diet with cooked foods and avoid raw or undercooked items.

Safe Food Storage: Properly store food in airtight containers and monitor refrigerator temperatures to prevent the growth of harmful bacteria.

Health Monitoring

Regular Screenings: Schedule regular health screenings to monitor overall health and detect any potential issues early.

Medical Care: Seek medical care promptly if experiencing symptoms associated with listeriosis or any other illness.

Preventing Listeriosis in Immunocompromised Individuals

Individuals with weakened immune systems, such as those undergoing chemotherapy or with chronic illnesses, face an elevated risk of listeriosis. Special precautions are necessary to protect their health.

Precautions and Practices

Strict Food Safety: Adhere strictly to food safety practices, including avoiding high-risk foods and ensuring proper cooking and storage.

Consult Healthcare Providers: Discuss specific dietary and health precautions with healthcare providers to tailor preventive measures to individual needs.

Support Systems

Family and Caregivers: Educate family members and caregivers about food safety practices and the importance of preventing listeriosis.

Healthcare Support: Regularly consult with healthcare professionals for advice and monitoring of health status.

CHAPTER 6

NAVIGATING LISTERIOSIS OUTBREAKS AND MANAGING SYMPTOMS

Introduction

Understanding how to navigate listeriosis outbreaks and manage symptoms is crucial for high-risk groups. This chapter delves into the steps to take during an outbreak, effective strategies for managing symptoms, and when to seek medical attention. By being informed and prepared, individuals can respond promptly to potential exposure and minimize the impact of listeriosis.

Identifying and Responding to an Outbreak

Listeriosis outbreaks can occur in various settings, including community settings, healthcare facilities, and food production environments. Being able to recognize an outbreak and respond effectively is key to managing risk.

Recognizing an Outbreak

Outbreak Indicators: Outbreaks may be identified through public health reports, increased cases of listeriosis in specific areas, or contamination reports linked to food products. Pay attention to alerts from health authorities and food safety organizations.

Symptoms Monitoring: Be aware of the symptoms of listeriosis, including fever, muscle aches, nausea, vomiting, and diarrhea. Symptoms may vary depending on the individual's age and health status.

Immediate Actions During an Outbreak

Avoiding Contaminated Products: Follow public health advisories and avoid consuming any foods or products that are linked to the outbreak. This may involve discarding recalled items and avoiding specific brands or products.

Enhancing Food Safety Measures: Increase vigilance in food safety practices, including thorough cooking, proper storage, and avoidance of high-risk foods. Ensure that all kitchen practices are up-to-date and rigorous.

Communicating with Health Authorities

Reporting Symptoms: If you suspect exposure or experience symptoms of listeriosis, contact healthcare providers and report your symptoms. Provide information about potential exposure sources and any recent food consumption.

Following Guidance: Adhere to guidance provided by health authorities regarding testing, treatment, and preventive measures. Keep informed about the status of the outbreak and any additional recommendations.

Managing Symptoms of Listeriosis

Early management of listeriosis symptoms can improve outcomes and prevent complications. This section focuses on the steps to take when symptoms are present and how to manage them effectively.

Recognizing Symptoms

Common Symptoms: Symptoms of listeriosis typically include fever, muscle aches, nausea, vomiting, and diarrhea. In more severe cases, individuals may experience headache, stiff neck, confusion, loss of balance, or convulsions.

Symptom Variation: Symptoms may vary depending on the individual's health status and age. Pregnant women, the elderly, and immunocompromised individuals may experience more severe symptoms.

Immediate Care for Symptoms

Rest and Hydration: Rest is essential when experiencing symptoms of listeriosis. Ensure adequate hydration by drinking fluids to prevent dehydration, especially if experiencing vomiting or diarrhea.

Over-the-Counter Medications: For mild symptoms, over-the-counter medications such as anti-nausea or anti-diarrheal medications may provide relief. However, consult a healthcare provider before using these medications, especially if symptoms are severe.

Seeking Medical Attention

When to See a doctor: Seek medical attention if symptoms are severe, persistent, or worsening. Immediate medical care is crucial for high-risk individuals, including pregnant women, the elderly, and those with compromised immune systems.

Diagnostic Tests: Healthcare providers may recommend diagnostic tests, such as blood tests, stool cultures, or lumbar punctures, to confirm the presence of Listeria monocytogenes and assess the extent of the infection.

Treatment Options for Listeriosis

Effective treatment of listeriosis typically involves antibiotics, and the approach may vary depending on the severity of the infection and the patient's health status.

Antibiotic Therapy

Common Antibiotics: The primary treatment for listeriosis is antibiotic therapy. Commonly used antibiotics include ampicillin and penicillin. In cases of severe infection or allergy to penicillin, alternative antibiotics such as trimethoprim-sulfamethoxazole may be prescribed.

Treatment Duration: The duration of antibiotic therapy varies depending on the severity of the infection and the patient's response to treatment. Follow healthcare provider instructions regarding the full course of antibiotics.

Specialized Care

Hospitalization: Severe cases of listeriosis, particularly those involving complications or high-risk groups, may require hospitalization. Hospital care may include intravenous antibiotics, supportive care, and monitoring for complications.

Monitoring and Follow-Up: Regular follow-up appointments may be necessary to monitor recovery progress and ensure that the infection has been effectively treated.

Managing Listeriosis in High-Risk Populations

For high-risk populations, including pregnant women, the elderly, and those with compromised immune systems, additional precautions and management strategies are essential.

Pregnant Women

Early Treatment: Prompt treatment with antibiotics is crucial for pregnant women diagnosed with listeriosis to prevent complications for both the mother and the unborn child.

Monitoring the Baby: After treatment, additional monitoring may be required to assess the health of the baby, including ultrasounds and other diagnostic tests.

Elderly Individuals

Close Monitoring: Elderly individuals with listeriosis may require more intensive monitoring and care due to potential complications and coexisting health conditions.

Supportive Care: Supportive care, including managing symptoms and addressing any complications, is vital for recovery.

Immunocompromised Individuals

Individualized Treatment: Treatment for immunocompromised individuals may require adjustments based on their specific health conditions and the extent of immune system compromise.

Ongoing Medical Supervision: Regular medical supervision and follow-up care are essential for managing listeriosis and preventing complications.

Preventive Measures After Exposure

Taking preventive measures after potential exposure to Listeria monocytogenes can reduce the risk of developing listeriosis.

Immediate Actions

Disposal of Contaminated Food: Discard any food items that may have been contaminated and follow food safety guidelines to prevent further exposure.

Enhanced Hygiene Practices: Increase hygiene practices, including thorough handwashing and cleaning of kitchen surfaces, to reduce the risk of secondary contamination.

Monitoring for Symptoms

Symptom Watch: Monitor for symptoms of listeriosis for several days following potential exposure. If symptoms develop, seek medical attention promptly.

Health Monitoring: For high-risk individuals, regular health monitoring and early consultation with healthcare providers are crucial to managing potential infections.

Support and Resources

Accessing support and resources can provide valuable assistance for individuals affected by listeriosis or those at risk.

Support Groups

Online Forums: Join online forums or support groups for individuals affected by listeriosis or high-risk groups. Sharing experiences and receiving support can be beneficial.

Community Organizations: Engage with community organizations that offer resources and support for individuals managing listeriosis and related health concerns.

Healthcare Resources

Healthcare Providers: Maintain regular contact with healthcare providers for advice, treatment, and monitoring related to listeriosis.

Public Health Agencies: Stay informed through public health agencies, such as the CDC and local health departments, for updates on outbreaks, preventive measures, and treatment options.

Chapter 7 Building a Listeria-Free Environment: Best Practices for Homes and Institutions

Introduction

Creating a listeria-free environment is essential for preventing listeriosis, especially in high-risk groups. This chapter explores best practices for maintaining cleanliness and safety in both residential and institutional settings. We'll examine how to implement effective food safety protocols, establish robust cleaning routines, and create a culture of awareness to minimize the risk of Listeria monocytogenes contamination.

Understanding the Risks

Sources of Listeria Monocytogenes

Contaminated Food Products: Listeria monocytogenes can be found in a variety of foods, particularly those that are not cooked or processed properly. High-risk foods include deli meats, unpasteurized dairy products, and certain ready-to-eat foods.

Environmental Contamination: The bacterium can also be present in soil, water, and animal feces. It can contaminate food through contact with these environmental sources, especially if proper sanitation practices are not followed.

Cross-Contamination: Listeria can spread from contaminated surfaces, utensils, or hands to other foods, creating a risk of infection if these foods are not properly handled or cooked.

High-Risk Environments

Healthcare Facilities: Hospitals and nursing homes often care for individuals with weakened immune systems, making these settings particularly vulnerable to outbreaks of listeriosis.

Food Processing Plants: These facilities can be hotspots for Listeria contamination due to the large volumes of food processed and the complex, often inadequate sanitation measures.

Households with Vulnerable Individuals: Homes with pregnant women, the elderly, or immunocompromised individuals require heightened vigilance in food safety and hygiene.

Best Practices for Food Safety

Proper Food Handling

Thorough Cooking: Cook all meats, poultry, and seafood to the recommended internal temperatures to kill any potential Listeria bacteria. Use a food thermometer to ensure that foods reach the appropriate temperature.

Safe Food Storage: Store perishable foods in the refrigerator at or below 40°F (4°C). Ensure that raw meats are kept separate from ready-to-eat foods to prevent cross-contamination.

Correct Thawing Methods: Thaw frozen foods in the refrigerator, under cold running water, or in the microwave, but never on the countertop. This prevents bacteria from multiplying at room temperature.

Avoiding High-Risk Foods

Unpasteurized Products: Avoid consuming unpasteurized milk and dairy products, as pasteurization kills harmful bacteria including Listeria.

Processed Meats: If consuming deli meats or hot dogs, ensure they are heated to steaming hot before eating. This can kill any Listeria bacteria present.

Ready-to-Eat Foods: For vulnerable populations, avoid ready-to-eat foods that have been recalled or are associated with recent outbreaks.

Implementing Effective Cleaning and Sanitation Protocols

Kitchen Hygiene

Regular Cleaning: Clean kitchen surfaces, utensils, and appliances regularly using hot, soapy water. Pay special attention to cutting boards, countertops, and refrigerator shelves.

Disinfecting: Use a disinfectant or a solution of bleach and water to sanitize surfaces that come into contact with raw foods. Follow manufacturer instructions for proper dilution and contact time.

Hand Hygiene: Wash hands with soap and water for at least 20 seconds before and after handling food, especially raw meats.

Encourage everyone in the household to practice good hand hygiene.

Maintaining a Clean Environment

Proper Waste Management: Dispose of food waste and packaging promptly and properly. Use sealed garbage containers and clean them regularly to prevent attracting pests.

Cleaning Schedules: Establish a routine cleaning schedule for kitchen and dining areas. Regularly clean high-touch areas such as refrigerator handles, cabinet knobs, and light switches.

Managing Spills: Clean up spills and crumbs immediately to prevent contamination. Use paper towels or cloths designated for cleaning, and ensure they are washed frequently.

Safeguarding Institutions

Food Service Facilities

Staff Training: Train food handlers on food safety practices, including proper cooking temperatures, cross-contamination prevention, and personal hygiene.

Sanitation Practices: Implement and monitor strict sanitation protocols, including regular cleaning and disinfecting of kitchen equipment, surfaces, and utensils.

Regular Inspections: Conduct regular inspections of food storage and preparation areas to ensure compliance with food safety standards and identify potential risks.

Healthcare and Institutional Settings

Infection Control: Establish infection control measures to prevent the spread of Listeria and other pathogens. This includes proper hand hygiene, use of personal protective equipment, and thorough cleaning of patient areas.

Patient Food Safety: For institutions providing food to patients, ensure that food is prepared, stored, and served following strict food safety guidelines to protect vulnerable individuals.

Environmental Monitoring: Regularly monitor and test environments for potential contamination sources. Implement corrective actions based on findings to maintain a safe environment.

Creating a Culture of Awareness

Educating Individuals

Public Awareness Campaigns: Participate in or promote public awareness campaigns that highlight the importance of food safety and hygiene in preventing listeriosis.

Community Engagement: Engage with community organizations, schools, and local groups to spread knowledge about safe food practices and listeriosis prevention.

Training and Resources

Training Programs: Develop and provide training programs for both staff and the public on food safety, including the risks of Listeria and best practices for prevention.

Educational Materials: Provide accessible educational materials, such as pamphlets, posters, and online resources, to inform individuals about listeriosis and how to prevent it.

Monitoring and Evaluation

Assessing Effectiveness

Regular Reviews: Regularly review and update food safety and sanitation protocols to ensure they remain effective and aligned with current guidelines.

Feedback Mechanisms: Implement feedback mechanisms to gather insights from staff and individuals about the effectiveness of current practices and identify areas for improvement.

Addressing Challenges

Adapting to Changes: Stay informed about new research and developments related to Listeria and food safety. Adapt practices and protocols as needed to address emerging challenges.

Continuous Improvement: Foster a culture of continuous improvement by regularly evaluating and enhancing food safety and sanitation practices based on feedback and new information.

Appendices

Glossary of Terms

Bacteria: Microorganisms that can cause disease, including foodborne illnesses like listeriosis.

Cross-Contamination: The transfer of harmful bacteria from one food product to another, often through improper handling or sanitation.

Deli Meats: Processed meats such as ham, turkey, and salami that are often found at delis or in pre-packaged forms.

Foodborne Illness: Illness caused by consuming contaminated food or beverages.

Listeria Monocytogenes: A type of bacteria that causes listeriosis, particularly dangerous to pregnant women, the elderly, and immunocompromised individuals.

Listeriosis: An infection caused by the Listeria monocytogenes bacteria, often contracted through contaminated food.

Pasteurization: A process of heating food and beverages to a specific temperature for a set period to kill harmful bacteria.

Perishable Foods: Foods that spoil quickly if not stored properly, such as dairy products, meats, and some fruits and vegetables.

Ready-to-Eat Foods: Foods that do not require further cooking before consumption, such as salads, cold cuts, and pre-cooked meals.

Sanitation: The practice of keeping areas clean and free from harmful bacteria and viruses to prevent illness.

Frequently Asked Questions

Q: What is listeriosis and how can I prevent it?

A: Listeriosis is an infection caused by the Listeria monocytogenes bacteria. To prevent it, avoid high-risk foods, practice good hygiene, cook foods thoroughly, and store foods at the correct temperatures.

Q: Which foods are most likely to be contaminated with Listeria?

A: Foods most likely to be contaminated include unpasteurized dairy products, deli meats, hot dogs, smoked seafood, and certain ready-to-eat foods.

Q: How can pregnant women reduce the risk of listeriosis?

A: Pregnant women should avoid unpasteurized dairy products, deli meats unless heated until steaming hot, and any recalled or high-risk foods. Practicing good food hygiene and cooking foods thoroughly are also essential.

Q: What should I do if I think I have eaten contaminated food?

A: If you suspect you have eaten contaminated food and experience symptoms such as fever, muscle aches, nausea, or diarrhea, seek medical attention immediately.

Q: Can Listeria be killed by cooking?

A: Yes, Listeria can be killed by cooking foods to the appropriate temperatures. Use a food thermometer to ensure meats, poultry, and seafood are cooked thoroughly.

Q: How should I clean my kitchen to prevent Listeria contamination?

A: Clean all surfaces, utensils, and cutting boards with hot, soapy water. Sanitize with a solution of bleach and water. Keep raw and cooked foods separate to avoid cross-contamination.

Q: Are there special precautions for the elderly or immunocompromised individuals?

A: Yes, individuals in these groups should be extra vigilant with food safety, avoiding high-risk foods, ensuring thorough cooking, and maintaining strict hygiene practices.

Sample Meal Plans

Meal Plan for Pregnant Women

Breakfast:

- Scrambled eggs with spinach and cheese (made with pasteurized cheese)
- Whole grain toast
- Fresh fruit salad

- Pasteurized orange juice

Lunch:

- Grilled chicken salad with mixed greens, tomatoes, and cucumbers (ensure all vegetables are washed thoroughly)
- Whole wheat roll
- Yogurt (pasteurized)

Dinner:

- Baked salmon with steamed broccoli and quinoa
- Mixed berry dessert with a dollop of pasteurized whipped cream

Snacks:

- Carrot sticks with hummus
- Apple slices with peanut butter

Meal Plan for the Elderly

Breakfast:

- Oatmeal with sliced bananas and a sprinkle of cinnamon
- Whole grain toast with avocado spread
- Pasteurized milk

Lunch:

- Turkey and cheese sandwich on whole grain bread (ensure turkey is heated until steaming)
- Side of carrot and celery sticks
- Pear

Dinner:

- Roast beef with sweet potatoes and green beans
- Mixed green salad with vinaigrette

Snacks:

- Cottage cheese (pasteurized) with pineapple chunks
- Whole grain crackers with cheese

Meal Plan for Immunocompromised Individuals

Breakfast:

- Greek yogurt (pasteurized) with honey and berries
- Whole grain cereal with pasteurized milk

Lunch:

- Lentil soup with a side of whole grain bread
- Apple slices

Dinner:

- Grilled chicken breast with brown rice and sautéed vegetables
- Fresh fruit salad

Snacks:

- Almonds and dried cranberries
- Sliced cucumbers with cream cheese

Contact Information for Health Agencies

Centers for Disease Control and Prevention (CDC)

- Website: www.cdc.gov
- Phone: 1-800-CDC-INFO (1-800-232-4636)
- Address: 1600 Clifton Road, Atlanta, GA 30329, USA

Food and Drug Administration (FDA)

- Website: www.fda.gov
- Phone: 1-888-INFO-FDA (1-888-463-6332)
- Address: 10903 New Hampshire Avenue, Silver Spring, MD 20993, USA

United States Department of Agriculture (USDA)

Website: www.usda.gov
Phone: 1-202-720-2791
Address: 1400 Independence Avenue, SW, Washington, D.C. 20250, USA

World Health Organization (WHO)

Website: www.who.int
Phone: +41-22-7912111
Address: Avenue Appia 20, 1211 Geneva 27, Switzerland

Further Reading and References

Centers for Disease Control and Prevention (CDC). "Listeria (Listeriosis)." Available at: https://www.cdc.gov/listeria/index.html

Food and Drug Administration (FDA). "Food Safety for Moms-to-Be." Available at: https://www.fda.gov/food/people-risk-foodborne-illness/food-safety-moms-be

United States Department of Agriculture (USDA). "Food Safety and Inspection Service." Available at: https://www.fsis.usda.gov/

World Health Organization (WHO). "Listeriosis." Available at: https://www.who.int/news-room/fact-sheets/detail/listeriosis

Mayo Clinic. "Listeria Infection (Listeriosis)." Available at: https://www.mayoclinic.org/diseases-conditions/listeria-infection/symptoms-causes/syc-20355269

www.ingramcontent.com/pod-product-compliance
Lightning Source LLC
Chambersburg PA
CBHW071937210526
45479CB00002B/724